Table of Contents

How To Read This Guide

- As you read through these chapters, you'll notice that there is medical and anatomical terminology. For those who aren't experienced in this type of language, don't fret! In the back of the book, you will find a glossary that lists and defines many of the words used.
- Every chapter has a list of various stretches with details on how to perform them correctly. You'll notice on every page, there will be a QR code. This code will link the stretch to a YouTube clip. This clip will show visual, step by step instructions (by yours truly) to make these stretches a breeze for you.
- Each chapter also has its list of muscles and muscle groups stretched. To keep you aware of where those muscles are located, and what they roughly look like, you'll see a section titled "Anatomy of a Stretcher" in the back of the book.
- There is no shame in re-reading instructions or starting with one stretch at a time. As the saying goes, practice makes perfect.

Chapter I: Why Stretching Matters

Stretching is essential for achieving short— and long—term relief after engaging in both physical and sedentary activities.

It helps us preserve mobility and reduce the risk of future injuries.

Let's be honest, we've all let out that groan of alleviation when we've stretched our necks and backs out after a long day, as we should!

Stress relief is also a huge additional benefit from our stretching efforts, so what's there to lose?

In this guide, I'll walk you through what to do, when to do it, and show you how important it all is for your health.

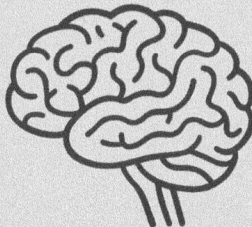

Chapter 2:
Stretching Do's and Don'ts

Static vs Dynamic Stretching (Let's compare these).

Static (or sustained) stretching is the action of developing and improving flexibility without movement in multiple directions.

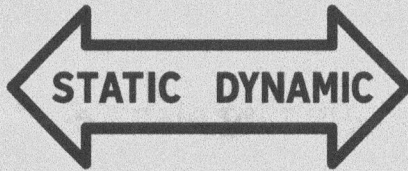

<------ STATIC   DYNAMIC ------>

Dynamic stretching is the action of developing and improving flexibility and mobility during involved movements in multiple directions.

Both have benefits, but in different ways.

Chapter 2:
Stretching Do's and Don'ts

Static Stretching, also known as Sustained Stretching, solely develops your flexibility and mobility in one direction for a period of time. The muscles, tendons, and ligaments in your body need to be able to move and depend on being flexible and mobile. Examples include toe touches, standing quad stretches, and similar movements.

Dynamic Stretching also develops your flexibility and mobility, but is more focused on repetitive movements in multiple directions. In other words, it is more active and can also help develop strength and coordination. Examples include leg swings, squats, lunges, arm circles, and similar movements.

Chapter 2:
Stretching Do's and Don'ts

The biggest question: When do I stretch?

This is definitely one of the age-old questions in the health (and chiropractic) community and I have the answer for you. Here it is: it all depends! Did you feel stiff waking up? Did you have a long day sitting down at work? Did you just run a marathon over the weekend? All jokes aside, everyone's flexibility, mobility, health, fitness, and stress levels are different. Even with my personal injury patients, I express greater caution due to their acute and subacute injuries.

Let's breakdown the scenarios...

Chapter 2:
Stretching Do's and Don'ts

<u>You're a stationary or semi-stationary worker</u>: look we've been there at some point in our lives where we're sitting in front of our computer monitors, focused on our tasks and paying almost no heed to the time that passes by. Sitting in one position for so long can increase stiffness and lead to dysfunction of your musculoskeletal system. Stretching is beneficial and generally low risk when working on it over time. We'll cover more of this in Chapter 4.

Chapter 2:
Stretching Do's and Don'ts

<u>You're a regular Joe-Schmo doing Joe-Schmo things (aka a regular person)</u>: you probably engage in a little bit of everything: from regular physical activity, to working at a desk, and maybe even being a parent. You're doing everything you can to be productive, but it can also gradually build pressure throughout your body. The soft and hard tissues in your body don't like this. In other words, fatigue can be a result of your efforts. Believe it or not, stretching is still beneficial.

Chapter 2:
Stretching Do's and Don'ts

<u>You're someone who just got injured</u>: this one is the trickiest of all scenarios and let me explain why. No two people are the same and no two injuries are the same. Soft tissue injuries and their symptoms can take anywhere from a week to months to recover. Different symptoms present such as local stiffness, local inflammation, muscle spasms, radiating pain, and decreased ROM (Range Of Motion). The body needs time and circulation of blood to heal soft tissue injuries. Once that is accomplished in an appropriate timeline and under the guidance of another doctor, then activities such as stretching can be introduced. I have always based my medical decision-making on introducing stretches to my patients based on a number of factors. When was their injury? What did they injure? How severe was the injury? Where is their current pain level right now? Are they experiencing any associated symptoms? How is their current range of motion? After I have these questions answered, I can designate a time to focus on flexibility and mobility.

Chapter 2:
Stretching Do's and Don'ts

<u>You're a parent</u>: and your bodies need tender loving care too. You're cooking, cleaning, driving, lifting, bending, sitting, standing, and god knows whatever else I missed. The point is that you're handling a high physical load and pushing through pain and stiffness to take care of your family. It's very difficult to find a second to even breathe. However, if you have as little as 3 minutes to spare, the difference stretching can make in your life is significant.

Chapter 2:
Stretching Do's and Don'ts

The next big question: When is not a good time to stretch?

As I've mentioned before, every situation is different. Injury vs no injury. Workplace ergonomics vs parental responsibilities. There is a mix of it all. However, there are some general contraindications to stretching...

- Severe or significant injury causing immobility
- Spinal and extra-spinal fractures
- Acute inflammation
- Presence of prominent bone spurs
- Joint instability
- Soft tissue trauma (hematomas, significant ecchymosis, severe lacerations or abrasions, etc.)

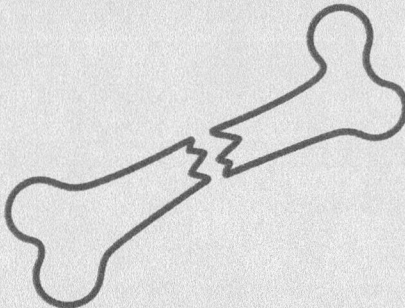

Chapter 2:
Stretching Do's and Don'ts

Frequency, Duration, and Safety Tips:

How often should you stretch and for how long?

Everyday. There are 24 hours, 1440 minutes, and 86,400 seconds in a day. Stretching is low risk (when warranted) and as you can see, it only takes a small amount of time in the day. With the routines that I'm going to show in the later chapters, it will take no longer than 15 minutes to stretch your entire body as a pre-/post- workout routine or to incorporate it into your daily routine. A static and dynamic protocol will be established.

Chapter 2:
Stretching Do's and Don'ts

Let's talk Safety Tips:
- Be motivated to stretch— without it, your results will fall flat and these routines will feel underwhelming.
- Have an open area that is free of any obstructions. You want to avoid anything that limits freedom of movement.
- In terms of breathing, it is strongly advisable to inhale slowly before performing the stretch and slowly exhaling while performing the stretch. Never, ever, ever hold in your breath while stretching. Increased pressure in your chest and abdomen can lead to discomfort and possible injury.

Chapter 2:
Stretching Do's and Don'ts

- Do not perform stretching when you are under the influence of alcohol or hallucinogenic drugs.
- Do not perform any stretches according to the prior contraindications as listed.
- As a general rule of thumb regarding posture, don't put your spine in a compromising position that hyper-mobilizes it. In other words, don't "push through".

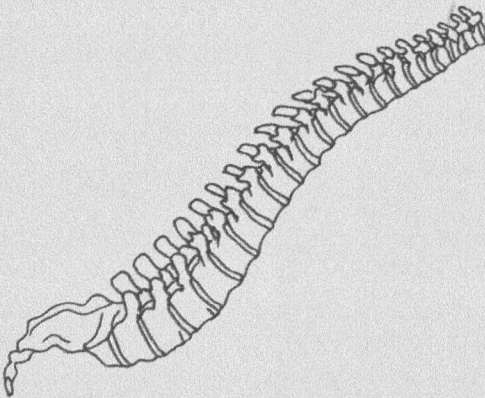

Chapter 3:
Morning Mobilizer

When waking up in the morning you can feel one of two things: plenty energized to take on the day or wake up full of stiffness. Many of my patients assign this experience to "sleeping wrong" and nothing more. If you fall in this category, trust me there is still hope. I'm going to run through some stretches that are quick, efficient, and easy to fit into your morning routine. The beauty of it is that you can do whatever you'd like in that moment. In this chapter, I'll be covering the neck (cervical spine), middle back (thoracic spine), lower back (lumbar spine), shoulders, hips, and ankles.

What you'll need: you, an open space, and just a bit of time.

General directions: 1-3 sets, 5-10 repetitions, and holding for 2-3 seconds.

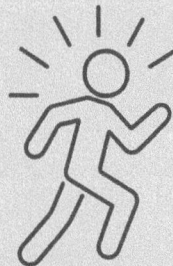

Chapter 3:
Morning Mobilizer

- Spine:
  - Static (Sustained)
    - Cervical
      - -Flexion
      - -Extension
      - -Lateral Flexion (left and right)
      - -Rotation (left and right)
      - -Major muscles stretched: Trapezius, SCM (sternocleidomastoids), Levator Scapulae, and Cervical Erector Spinae Muscle Groups.
    - Thoracic
      - -Flexion
      - -Extension
      - -Lateral Flexion (left and right)
      - -Rotation (left and right)
      - -Major muscles stretched: Trapezius, Latissimus Dorsi, Levator Scapulae, Rhomboids, and Thoracic Erector Spinae Muscle Groups.
    - Lumbar
      - -Flexion
      - -Extension
      - -Lateral Flexion (left and right)
      - -Rotation (left and right)
      - -Major muscles stretched: Lumbar Erector Spinae Muscle Groups, Obliques, and Quadratus Lumborum.

(Cervical)   (Thoracic)   (Lumbar)

Chapter 3:
Morning Mobilizer

○ Combined Cervical Range of Motion movement:
  ▪ Standing, sitting, or lying down. Lying down isn't ideal due to limited freedom of movement. Four different quadrants where combined movement will be performed:
    -Lower Left Quadrant: Flexion, Left Rotation, and Left Lateral Flexion.
    -Lower Right Quadrant: Flexion, Right Rotation, and Right Lateral Flexion.
    -Upper Left Quadrant: Extension, Left Rotation, and Left Lateral Flexion.
    -Upper Right Quadrant: Extension, Right Rotation, and Right Lateral Flexion.
    -Major muscles stretched: Trapezius, SCM (sternocleidomastoids), Levator Scapulae, and Cervical Erector Spinae Muscle Groups.
    -Cervical Ranges of Motion performed: Flexion, Extension, Lateral Flexion (left and right), and Rotation (left and right).

(Your visual field)

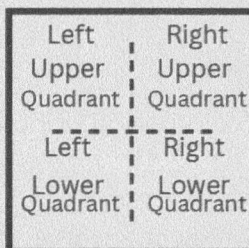

Left Upper Quadrant	Right Upper Quadrant
Left Lower Quadrant	Right Lower Quadrant

Chapter 3:
Morning Mobilizer

○ Combined Thoracic Range of Motion movement:
  ▪ Standing or sitting. Lying down isn't ideal due to limited freedom of movement. Four different quadrants where combined movement will be performed:
    -Lower Left Quadrant: Flexion, Left Rotation, and Left Lateral Flexion.
    -Lower Right Quadrant: Flexion, Right Rotation, and Right Lateral Flexion.
    -Upper Left Quadrant: Extension, Left Rotation, and Left Lateral Flexion.
    -Upper Right Quadrant: Extension, Right Rotation, and Right Lateral Flexion.
    -Major muscles stretched: Latissimus Dorsi, Rhomboids, Trapezius, Serratus Posterior Superior and Inferior, Thoracic Erector Spinae Muscle Groups.
    -Thoracic Ranges of Motion performed: Flexion, Extension, Lateral Flexion (left and right), and Rotation (left and right).

Chapter 3:
Morning Mobilizer

○ Combined Lumbar Range of Motion movement:

    ■ Lying down, standing, or sitting. Lying down is ideal since it takes pressure off the lumbar spine and lets the lower back muscles relax. Standing or sitting are also options, but this method would instead add pressure. Four different quadrants where combined movement will be performed:

       -Lower Left Quadrant: Flexion, Left Rotation, and Left Lateral Flexion.

       -Lower Right Quadrant: Flexion, Right Rotation, and Right Lateral Flexion.

       -Upper Left Quadrant: Extension, Left Rotation, and Left Lateral Flexion.

       -Upper Right Quadrant: Extension, Right Rotation, and Right Lateral Flexion.

       -Major muscles stretched: Latissimus Dorsi, Thoracolumbar Fascia (not a muscle, but is a contributor to stiffness in the lower back), Quadratus Lumborum, and Erector Spinae Muscle Groups.

       -Lumbar Ranges of Motion performed: Flexion, Extension, Lateral Flexion (left and right), and Rotation (left and right).

Chapter 3:
Morning Mobilizer

- **Shoulders:**
  - **Static (Sustained):**
    - **Flexion**
    - **Extension**
    - **Internal Rotation**
    - **External Rotation**
    - **Abduction**
    - **Adduction**

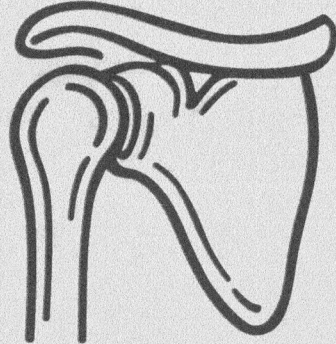

  - **Combined Shoulder Range of Motion movement:**
    - **Standing, interlocking fingers, turning them outwards, and raising them above your head. Hold position, then switch to the second part of the stretch. Standing, hands and arms behind, interlocking your fingers, bringing your chest out, and pulling arms down (Handcuff position).**
    - **Major muscles stretched: Rotator Cuff Muscles, Pectoralis Major, Pectoralis Minor, Trapezius, and Latissimus Dorsi muscles.**
    - **Shoulder Ranges of Motion performed: Flexion, Extension, Abduction, Adduction, Internal Rotation, and External Rotation.**

(Sustained)   (Combined)

Chapter 3:
Morning Mobilizer

- Hips:
  - Static (Sustained):
    - Flexion
    - Extension
    - Internal Rotation
    - External Rotation
    - Abduction
    - Adduction

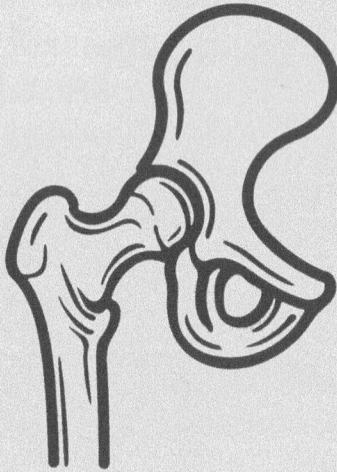

Chapter 3:
Morning Mobilizer

○ Combined Hip Range of Motion movement:
- ■ Hip CARs (Controlled Articular Rotations)
- -The ideal position for this would be standing. Lying down or sitting would limit freedom of movement in this stretch. Stand beside a wall for balance with feet shoulder-width apart. Keep one leg planted. Lift the opposite knee, crossing it over the standing leg. Rotate the lifted leg outward (heel in, knee out), then inward (heel down, knee in). Turn the knee out to the side, then rotate it inward across your body. Return to the start with a slight knee bend and repeat.
- -Major muscles stretched: Gluteus Maximus, Quadriceps, and Hamstring muscles.
- -Hip Ranges of Motion performed: Flexion, Extension, Abduction, Adduction, Internal Rotation, and External Rotation.

Chapter 3:
Morning Mobilizer

- Ankles:
  - Static (Sustained):
    - Dorsiflexion
    - Plantar flexion
    - Inversion
    - Eversion

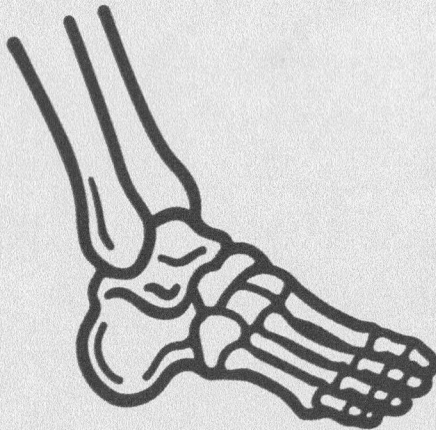

Chapter 3:
Morning Mobilizer

○ Combined Ankle Range of Motion movement:
- Lying down or sitting. Lying down is ideal since it takes pressure off the ankle joints and allows more freedom of movement. Begin by bending both knees on the flat surface you are lying on. Extend the desired leg and foot out so that the ankle is able to move freely in the air. Then, perform movements in the corresponding four quadrants:
  - -dorsiflexion + inversion
  - -dorsiflexion + eversion
  - -plantar flexion + inversion
  - -plantar flexion + eversion
  - -Major muscles stretched: Gastrocnemius (calf muscles), Soleus, Tibialis Anterior, and Tibialis Posterior.
  - -Ankle Ranges of Motion performed: Dorsiflexion, Plantar flexion, Inversion, and Eversion.

Chapter 3:
Morning Mobilizer

Keep In Mind: This morning mobilizer is designed to take 5 minutes or less. This all depends on how much you stretch in general and how much time you have. There is no need to complete the entire motion of a stretch if you're unable to do it. This is why we work on it in the first place.

Chapter 4:
Desk Relief Routine

You wake up, get ready for work, and hopefully with the sufficient time of sleep you received, you're ready to take on the day. Although things may seem fine when you're getting settled into the office for the first few hours, but you slowly notice how tight and stiff you feel in the latter half of the work day. To counteract this, here's a targeted routine designed for desk-bound warriors. In this chapter, I'll be covering the neck (cervical spine), lower back (lumbar spine), shoulders, and wrists.

What you'll need: you, ideally an open space, and just a bit of time. It can even be done in the cubicle you work in. Just be mindful of what is around you.

General directions: 1-3 sets, 5-10 repetitions, holding for 2-3 seconds. If time is a constraint, try reducing to 1 set, halving the reps, and holding each stretch for 1–2 seconds.

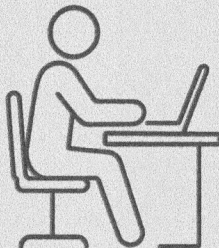

Chapter 4:
Desk Relief Routine

- Spine:
  - Static (Sustained):
    - Cervical
      -Flexion
      -Extension
      -Lateral Flexion (left and right)
      -Rotation (left and right)
      -Major muscles stretched: Trapezius, SCM (sternocleidomastoids), Levator Scapulae, and Cervical Erector Spinae Muscle Groups.
    - Lumbar
      -Flexion
      -Extension
      -Lateral Flexion (left and right)
      -Rotation (left and right)
      -Major muscles stretched: Lumbar Erector Spinae Muscle Groups, Obliques, and Quadratus Lumborum.

(Cervical)   (Lumbar)

Chapter 4:
Desk Relief Routine

○ **Combined Cervical Range of Motion movement:**
  ▪ **Standing, sitting, or lying down. Four different quadrants where combined movement will be performed:**
  -**Lower Left Quadrant: Flexion, Left Rotation, and Left Lateral Flexion.**
  -**Lower Right Quadrant: Flexion, Right Rotation, and Right Lateral Flexion.**
  -**Upper Left Quadrant: Extension, Left Rotation, and Left Lateral Flexion.**
  -**Upper Right Quadrant: Extension, Right Rotation, and Right Lateral Flexion.**
  -**Major muscles stretched: Trapezius, SCM (sternocleidomastoids), Levator Scapulae, and Cervical Erector Spinae Muscle Gr oups.**
  -**Cervical Ranges of Motion performed: Flexion, Extension, Lateral Flexion (left and right), and Rotation (left and right).**

Chapter 4:
Desk Relief Routine

○ **Combined Lumbar Range of Motion movement:**
  ▪ Lying down or standing. Lying down is ideal since it takes pressure off the lumbar spine and lets the lower back muscles relax. Standing or sitting down would do the opposite. Four different quadrants where combined movement will be performed:
    -Lower Left Quadrant: Flexion, Left Rotation, and Left Lateral Flexion.
    -Lower Right Quadrant: Flexion, Right Rotation, and Right Lateral Flexion. -
    Upper Left Quadrant: Extension, Left Rotation, and Left Lateral Flexion.
    -Upper Right Quadrant: Extension, Right Rotation, and Right Lateral Flexion.
    -Major muscles stretched: Latissimus Dorsi, Thoracolumbar Fascia (not a muscle, but is a contributor to stiffness in the lower back), Quadratus Lumborum, and Erector Spinae Muscle Groups.
    -Lumbar Ranges of Motion performed: Flexion, Extension, Lateral Flexion (left and right), and Rotation (left and right).

Chapter 4:
Desk Relief Routine

- Shoulders:
  - Sustained:
    - Flexion
    - Extension
    - Internal Rotation
    - External Rotation
    - Abduction
    - Adduction
  - Combined Shoulder Range of Motion movement:
    - Standing, interlocking fingers, turning them outwards, and raising them above your head. Standing, hands, and arms behind, interlocking your fingers, bringing your chest out, and pulling arms down (Handcuff position).
    - Major muscles stretched: Rotator Cuff Muscles, Pectoralis Major, Pectoralis Minor, Trapezius, and Latissimus Dorsi muscles.
    - Shoulder Ranges of Motion performed: Flexion, Extension, Abduction, Adduction, Internal Rotation, and External Rotation.

(Sustained)

(Combined)

Chapter 4:
Desk Relief Routine

- Wrists:
  - Static (Sustained):
    - Flexion
    - Extension
    - Radial Deviation
    - Ulnar Deviation
    - Supination
    - Pronation

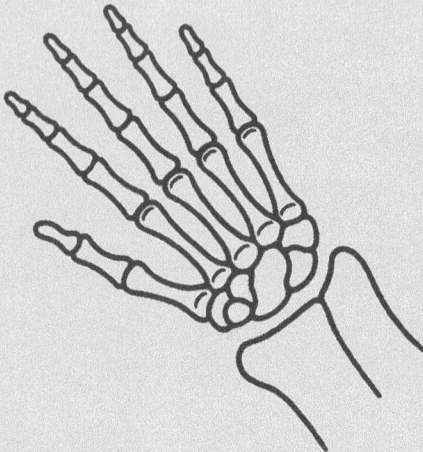

Chapter 4:
Desk Relief Routine

- Combined Wrist Range of Motion movement:
  - Sitting, standing, or lying down. Either position is ideal since the wrist joint has more freedom of movement than the ankle and the shoulder.
    -In the first combined movement, start with palms facing up, twist your forearm upwards to follow your palm, bend your open palm towards you and then bend your wrist so your pinky moves closer to the inner part of your forearm.
    -In the second combined movement, start with the palm facing down, twist your forearm downwards to follow your palm, bend the back of your hand towards you and then bend your wrist so your thumb moves closer to the inner part of your forearm.
  - Major muscles stretched: Flexors and Extensors of the Forearm, and Biceps Brachii.
  - Wrist Ranges of Motion performed: Flexion, Extension, Supination, Pronation, Radial and Ulnar Deviation.
  - Keep in mind: A more open space is always better than just an office cubicle, but you are more than able to do with what you can.

Due to the intention of this guide being a quick reference, Chapters 3 and 4 can serve as a reference forthe Ranges of Motion of multiple parts of the body.

Chapter 5:
Post-Workout Recovery

Everyone's workouts are always going to be different. Everyone's strength (how much force muscles can generate) and power (the rate of which force is produced) are also different. However, the result is the same. After high physical activity, muscles will fatigue and soreness will result. As many people attribute muscle soreness to the production of lactic acid, it is actually due to micro-tears in the muscle! To many people, this may seem like a sign of a good workout. While stressed muscles can support growth, they still have their limits. What we're going to focus on here are static (sustained) stretches. In this chapter, I'll be covering the chest, hip flexors, quadriceps, hamstrings, calves, and gluteus muscles.

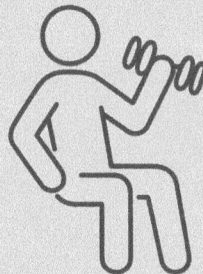

Chapter 5:
Post-Workout Recovery

- What you'll need: you, a soft surface like a yoga mat (if possible), a wall, and 5-10 minutes depending on the muscle groups exercised.
- General directions: 1-3 sets, 5-10 repetitions, and holding for 2-3 seconds.

Chapter 5:
Post-Workout Recovery

- Chest:
  - Static (Sustained):
    - Wall Stretch
      - The ideal position would be standing next to a wall. Have the left or right side of your body near the wall. This will be the side you would like to stretch. Then, place your hand (closest to the wall) on the wall itself, keeping it in a fixed position and walking slowly forward. You will feel the stretch in your upper chest and front of your shoulder.
      - Major muscles stretched: Pectoralis Major, Pectoralis Minor, and Anterior Head of Deltoid.

- Tip: Both of your pectoral (chest) muscles attach to the humerus (upper arm), so to feel the stretch in this area of the upper arm as well is normal.

Chapter 5:
Post-Workout Recovery

- Quads:
  - Static (Sustained):
    - Standing (or Side Lying) Quad Stretch
      -The ideal position would be standing or lying down. Sitting down would prevent freedom of movement. While standing, bend the knee of the leg you want to stretch, and use your hand of the same side to grasp and hold your ankle. The heel of the bent leg will touch the buttock of the same side. Side lying would be the same instructions, but the side that you're not stretching will be touching the floor.
      -Major muscles stretched: Quadriceps of the Upper Leg (Rectus Femoris, Vastus Medialis, Vastus Lateralis, and Vastus Intermedius.

- Tip: It is better to perform this stretch (and generally all stretches) slowly and not quickly. If you see that you're having issues trying to balance while standing, use a wall for support.

Chapter 5:
Post-Workout Recovery

- Hamstrings
  - Static (Sustained):
    - Sitting Hamstring Stretch (aka Toe Touch Stretch)
      -The ideal position would be sitting preferably on yoga mat. Sitting on a mat, extend the leg of the desired side you want to stretch out, bend the other leg in, and bend down slowly as if to touch your toes. Make sure to repeat on the opposite leg.
      -Muscles stretched: Hamstrings (Semitendinosus, Semimembranosus, Biceps Femoris), Adductor Magnus, Gracilis, and Gluteus Maximus.

- Tip: It is better to perform this stretch (and generally all stretches) slowly and not quickly. If you are unable to touch your toes, start by extending the knee first and then gradually work your way down from there. You can work your way down progressively in the same session or overtime. Remember, baby steps!

Chapter 5:
Post-Workout Recovery

- Calves
  - Static (Sustained):
    - Calf Wall Stretch
      - -The ideal position would be standing. First, face the wall. Next, put one leg out and put the tip of your foot (forefoot) against the wall. Last, lean into the wall while keeping the forefoot against the wall. Make sure to repeat on the opposite calf.
      - -Major muscles stretched: Gastrocnemius, Soleus, and Tibialis Posterior.

- Tip: Please perform this stretch slowly as calf muscles are notoriously very tight.

Chapter 5:
Post-Workout Recovery

- Glutes and Hip Flexors (also quads and hamstrings)
  - Static (Sustained):
    - One-Legged Lunge Stretch
      -The ideal position for this is to be on a yoga mat, on your knees, one leg back extended (knee and leg behind you) and the other leg forward, bent at the knee, and at the hip. Once you're in this position, lean forward into the bent leg.
      -Major muscles stretched: Quadriceps and Hamstrings of the leg (Rectus Femoris, VastusMedialis,VastusLateralis, Vastus Intermedius, Semitendinosus, Semimembranosus and Biceps Femoris) Gracilis, Adductor Magnus, and Gluteus Maximus.

- Tip: As some would think that the bent leg is the only part you are stretching, but actually you are stretching out your glutes, hip flexors, quadriceps, and hamstrings all in one motion with this type of stretch.

Chapter 6:
Evening Wind Down

The day is finally coming to an end. You've had a long shift at work, scrambled to get home, had to make dinner, and take care of the home you left behind for so many hours. Believe me, I've been in your shoes before. It's physically taxing on your body and it needs time to recover. Let's focus on a routine (especially easy Yoga poses) that can help promote melatonin production by encouraging relaxation, reduce cortisol levels, and lead to an overall good night's sleep. In this chapter, I'll be covering the overall body.

What you'll need: you, an open space and to be in your bedroom.

General directions: 1-2 sets, 3-8 repetitions, holding for 5-10 seconds.

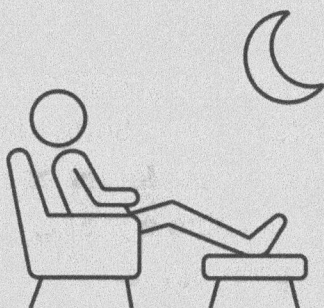

Chapter 6:
Evening Wind Down

- Overall Body
  - Static (Sustained):
    - Child's Pose (Balasana)
      - The ideal position is to be on a yoga mat on both knees. First, place your hands flat in front of you, about two feet away from your knees, feet pointing back, keep the neck and back parallel to the floor, and breathe in. As you exhale, bring your hips down to the floor while keeping your neck and back straight. Keep your hands firmly placed where they are in front of you and exhale. Finally, hold this position for 5-10 seconds. Repeat for another set. Maintain shallow breathing when you're holding the position downwards.
      - Major muscles stretched: Latissimus Dorsi, Thoracolumbar Fascia (not a muscle, but is a contributor to stiffness in the lower back), Quadratus Lumborum, Erector Spinae Muscle Groups,Quadriceps,andTrapeziusmuscles.

    - Tip: This stretch is a great way to stretch multiple parts of your body such as the neck, shoulders, mid back, lower back, quadriceps, and ankles. It is also a great, easy way to decompress your spine.

Chapter 6:
Evening Wind Down

- **Legs Up the Wall Pose (Viparita Karani)**
  -The ideal position is to be sitting in front of a
  wall. First, position yourself where your back
  is flat on the floor and legs (from butt to heel)
  are flat against the wall. Next, maintain this
  position and place your hands with palms
  open to the sides of your body. Finally, inhale
  and exhale slowly while holding the position.
  -Major muscles stretched: Thoracolumbar
  Fascia (not a muscle, but is a contributor to
  stiffness in the lower back), Quadratus
  Lumborum, Lumbar Erector Spinae Muscle
  Groups, Hamstrings (Semitendinosus,
  Semimembranosus, Biceps Femoris), Gracilis,
  and Adductor Magnus muscles.

- **Tip:** You can close your eyes during this pose as
  this may further help in relaxation. This pose is
  the exception to the 5-10 seconds rule. Instead,
  perform this position for 1-5 minutes.

Chapter 6:
Evening Wind Down

Warning: Being in this position for longer than 5 minutes may cause circulation issues to the lower extremities. If you have circulatory issues, cardiovascular conditions, or diabetes (whether controlled or uncontrolled) please express caution and consult your health provider.

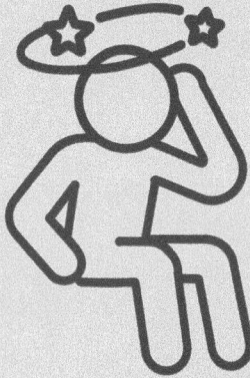

Chapter 6:
Evening Wind Down

- Neck Stretches
  - -The ideal position is to be sitting. This position allows greater freedom of movement and isolation of the neck muscles. Standing or lying down would do the opposite. Find a chair or a place to sit that has a back to it. Begin to follow the sustained ranges of motion listed in Chapters 3 and 4.
    - Sustained
      - Cervical
      - Flexion
      - Extension
      - Lateral Flexion (left and right)
      - Rotation (left and right)

Chapter 6:
Evening Wind Down

- Combined Cervical Range of Motion movement:
  - Four different quadrants where combined movement will be performed:
    - -Lower Left Quadrant: Flexion, Left Rotation, and Left Lateral Flexion.
    - -Lower Right Quadrant: Flexion, Right Rotation, and Right Lateral Flexion.
    - -Upper Left Quadrant: Extension, Left Rotation, and Left Lateral Flexion.
    - -Upper Right Quadrant: Extension, Right Rotation, and Right Lateral Flexion.
    - -Major muscles stretched: Trapezius, SCM (sternocleidomastoid), Levator Scapulae, and Cervical Erector Spinae Muscle Groups.
    - -Cervical Ranges of Motion performed: Flexion, Extension, Lateral Flexion (left and right), and Rotation (left and right).

- Tip: After a long day, this area may be tight, Go slowly, focusing on inhaling before starting and exhaling after performing the stretch.

Chapter 6:
Evening Wind Down

- **Corpse Pose (Savasana)**
  - The ideal position is to lie flat on your back on the floor, preferably on a yoga mat or soft surface. Next, place your arms will be to the sides of your body and your legs will be apart and straight. Finally, once in position, lie in this pose for 5 minutes or less, and to make sure that you are breathing in and out while performing the stretch.
  - Major muscles stretched: No muscles are technically stretched here. Instead, they are encouraged to be relaxed and release tension.

- **Tip:** This pose is also an exception to the 5-10 seconds rule. Instead, lie down in this position for 1-5 minutes. Set a timer on your phone or clock as this pose can be very relaxing!

Chapter 7:
Weekend Warrior Recovery

The weekend warrior has many definitions in this day and age, but it leads to only one type of individual. This individual is one who performs activities that are physically demanding on the weekends or in their free time. This would include the hikers, climbers, athletes, bicyclists, and gym goers. Sorry my fellow video gamers, you won't be counted in the list. For the groups of people I listed, you may be saying right now "Dr. Michael, I just did so much activity and exercise I can't possibly stretch out anything right now!". Let me go ahead and show you simple to perform stretches that require minimal effort. In this chapter, I'll be covering the middle back (thoracic spine), lower back (lumbar spine), shoulders, quadriceps, hamstrings, glutes, and hip flexor muscles. What you'll need: you and an open space. General directions: 1-2 sets, 3-8 repetitions, and holding for 5-10 seconds.

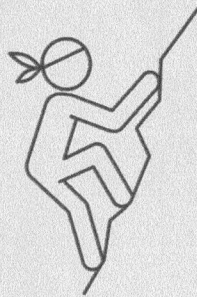

Chapter 7:
Weekend Warrior Recovery

- Pre-Activity (after a light warm-up)
  - Leg Swings
    - Dynamic
      - The ideal position for these would be to be standing next to a wall. Give yourself enough space where you can freely move your legs. First, you will position yourself with the desired leg to stretch away from the wall and the hand closest to the wall will be placed on the wall. Then, proceed to swing your legs forward and back at a moderate pace while keeping the leg as straight as possible. Perform this to the other leg.
      - Major muscles stretched: Quadriceps, Hamstrings, Gluteal muscles, and Hip Flexor muscles.

Chapter 7:
Weekend Warrior Recovery

- ○ Tip: To ensure you are feeling the stretch in the lower half of your body, make sure to maintain an upright posture of your neck, middle back and lower back.
- ○ Caution: There is no need to fully swing the legs to their limits. Performing this stretch to where you feel comfortable is enough.

Chapter 7:
Weekend Warrior Recovery

- Arm Circles
  - Dynamic
    - -The ideal position for this would be standing and far enough away from any obstructions (walls, standing objects, etc.). As the name already sounds, you're going to keep your fingers straight and proceed to move your entire arm in a circular fashion as if you're trying to draw a big circle to the side of you body. Proceed to do this at a moderate pace.
    - -Major muscles stretched: Deltoid, Pectoralis Muscles, Biceps Brachii, Triceps Brachii, Trapezius, and Latissimus Dorsi muscles.

- Tip: Since you are working more than one muscle group here, one of these is bound to be tight. Perform these slowly.

Chapter 7:
Weekend Warrior Recovery

○ **One-Legged Lunge Stretch**
- **Dynamic**
  -The ideal position for this is to be in a standing position or on a yoga mat. First, on your knees, extend one leg back (knee and leg behind you) and bring one leg forward bent at the knee and at the hip. Once you're in this position, lean yourself into the leg that is bent. Opposed to the static (sustained) version, you will perform this at a moderate pace and alternate legs.
  -Major muscles stretched: Quadriceps, Hamstrings, Glutes, and Hip Flexor muscles.

○ **Tip: As some would think that the bent leg is the only part you are stretching but actually you are stretching out your glutes, quadriceps, and hamstrings all in one motion with this type of stretch. Keep both hands on the floor to the sides of your body for added stabilization.**

Chapter 7:
Weekend Warrior Recovery

- Post-Activity
  - Lunging Hip Flexor Stretch
    - Static (Sustained)
      -The ideal position for this is to be in a standing position or on a yoga mat. First on your knees, one leg back extended and one leg forward bent at the knee and at the hip. Once you're in this position, place your hands on your hips, keep your back straight and bend the forward leg with the extended leg fixed in place. Once completed, perform the stretch to the other hip.

      -Major muscles stretched: Quadriceps, Hamstrings, Gluteal muscles, and Hip Flexor muscles.

  - Tip: Opposed to the One-Legged Lunge Stretch, this variation is focused on exclusively stretching the hip flexors (especially in the rear leg).

Chapter 7:
Weekend Warrior Recovery

○ Piriformis Stretch (aka Figure Four Stretch)
- ▪ Static (Sustained)
  - -The ideal position for this is to be seated or lying down. If <u>seated</u>, you'll first want to locate a chair that has a back and sit in an upright posture, with legs shoulder-width apart and feet touching the floor. Next, you will bring the leg and ankle— of the desired side you would like to stretch— to the top of your opposite thigh. This position will look like a "figure 4". Maintain this posture. Finally, you will lean forward and downwards as if you're trying to touch the floor. Perform this stretch to the other side. If <u>lying</u> on your back, you'll first want to find a floor that is soft and not uncomfortable. Next, you'll flex both knees and hips as if you're trying to sit in a chair. From here, bring the leg and ankle – of the desired side you would like to stretch— to the top of your opposite thigh. This position will look like a "figure 4". Finally, bring the leg that is under the crossed leg closer to your body.

Chapter 7:
Weekend Warrior Recovery

- Major muscles stretched: Latissimus Dorsi, Thoracolumbar Fascia (not a muscle, but is a contributor to stiffness in the lower back), Quadratus Lumborum, Erector Spinae Muscle Groups, Quadriceps, and Trapezius muscles.

○ Tip: This stretch is a great way to work on multiple parts of your body such as the neck, shoulders, mid back, lower back, quadriceps, and ankles. It is also a great, easy way to decompress your spine. You may feel soreness after performing this stretch due to all the physical activity you just performed so please take it slow.

Chapter 7:
Weekend Warrior Recovery

- Cross-Legged Side Bending Stretch
    - Static (Sustained)
        - The ideal position is to be next to a wall, feet shoulder-width apart, and the side of your body— the side you would like to stretch— facing away from the wall. First, place the hand closest to the wall onto the wall. Next, cross the foot and lower leg— that's facing away from the wall— onto the foot and lower leg closest to the wall. Then, lift the hand that's away from the wall into the air, arch it over your head, and (as close as possible) touch the wall. Finally, breathe slowly in and out while you sustain this stretch.

        - Major muscles stretched: Latissimus Dorsi, Thoracolumbar Fascia (not a muscle, but is a contributor to stiffness in the lower back), Quadratus Lumborum, and the sides of the Quadriceps muscles.

- Tip: This will require some balance to maintain this position. Make sure eyes are open for the entire duration of the stretch.

Chapter 8:
Travel Stretches

When people think of vacation the general thoughts are of beaches, big cities, eating at fancy restaurants, or physical activity that includes a lot of walking. Going on vacation is necessary for us working folk to relieve stress from the everyday activities we perform for 8 (or more) hours a day. Depending on your mode of travel, you'll be seated for extended periods of time and won't have easy access anywhere to stretch or walk around. I'll provide stretches you can perform before and during the trip. In this chapter, I'll be covering calves, hamstrings, hips, knees, ankles, glutes, neck (cervical spine), and shoulders.

What you'll need: you, an open space like a lobby, or waiting area and the seat that you're in. For safety, any variations on standing for these stretches will be excluded.

General directions: 3-5 sets, 5-10 repetitions, holding 3-5 seconds

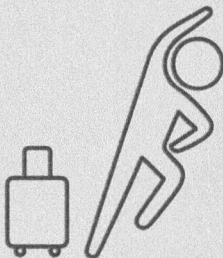

Chapter 8:
Travel Stretches

- Before the trip:
  - Static (Sustained)
    - Calf Stretch
      -The ideal position would be standing. First, find and face a wall or an elevated ledge. Next, put one leg out and put the tip of your foot (forefoot) against the wall or ledge. Last, slowly lean into the wall or ledge while keeping the forefoot against it. Make sure to repeat on the opposite calf.
      -Major muscles stretched: Gastrocnemius, Soleus, and Tibialis Posterior.

    - Tip: Perform this stretch slowly as calf muscles are notoriously very tight. For this stretch hold it for 3-5 seconds.

Chapter 8:
Travel Stretches

- **Toe Touch Stretch (aka Hamstring Stretch)**
  - The ideal position is to be standing or sitting on a flat surface. First, if <u>standing</u>, you will simply bend down slowly and attempt to touch your toes. If <u>sitting</u>, first extend your legs out onto the flat surface and attempt to touch your toes. Finally, while reaching the maximum range of this stretch, hold this position for 3-5 seconds.
  - Major muscles stretched: Lumbar Erector Spinae Muscle Groups, Quadratus Lumborum, Thoracolumbar fascia (not a muscle, but is a contributor to stiffness in the lower back) Hamstrings (Semitendinosus, Semimembranosus, Biceps Femoris) Gracilis, Adductor Magnus, and Gluteus Maximus.

- **Tip:** You do not need to touch your toes or go to maximum effort on this stretch. Remember you are doing 3-5 sets. A great place to start is halfway (knees) on the first set, then progressively stretch further with each ongoing set.

Chapter 8:
Travel Stretches

- **Figure Four Stretch (aka Piriformis stretch)**
  - The ideal position for this is to be seated or lying down. If <u>seated</u>, you'll first want to locate a chair that has a back and sit in an upright posture, with legs shoulder-width apart and feet touching the floor. Next, you will bring the leg and ankle— of the desired side you would like to stretch— to the top of your opposite thigh. This position will look like a "figure 4". Maintain this posture. Finally, you will lean forward and downwards as if you're trying to touch the floor. Perform this stretch to the other side. If <u>lying</u> on your back, you'll first want to find a floor that is soft and comfortable. Next, you'll flex both knees and hips as if you're trying to sit in a chair. From here, bring the leg and ankle— of the desired side you would like to stretch— to the top of your opposite thigh. This position will look like a "figure 4". Finally, bring the leg that is under the crossed leg closer to your body.

Chapter 8:
Travel Stretches

-Major muscles stretched: Gluteal muscles,
Tensor Fascia Latae (TFL), Upper Quadriceps,
and Piriformis muscles.

• Tip: These areas will be very sensitive so
please do this slowly and carefully.

Chapter 8:
Travel Stretches

- **During the trip:**
  - **Dynamic**
    - **Ankle Circles**
      - -The ideal position will be to be seated. You can be standing or lying down, but let's say you're in a moving vehicle, your safety is more important, space is limited, and balance may be required. First, you will lift the desired leg— that you would like to stretch —out in front of you. Next, pretend that with your toes you're going to draw a big circle in the air. Once completed with this side, alternate to the other ankle.
      - -Major muscles stretched: Gastrocnemius, Soleus, Tibialis Anterior, and Tibialis Posterior Muscles.

    - **Tip:** If space is limited in front of you, (damn you budget airlines!) then simply lift your knee if in the air and use that space where your feet were occupying.

Chapter 8:
Travel Stretches

- **Knee Hug**
  - The ideal position for this is seated. You can be standing or lying down, but let's say you're in a moving vehicle, your safety is more important space is limited and balance may be required. First, begin to lift the knee of the desired side you would like to stretch. Next, hold the knee tight to you as if you're giving it a hug and connect it to your chest. Finally, maintain this position and breathe. Once done with this side, alternate to the other knee.
  - Major muscles stretched: Lumbar Erector Spinae Muscles Groups, Quadratus Lumborum, Hamstrings (Semitendinosus, Semimembranosus, Biceps Femoris), and Quadriceps muscles.

- **Tip: A firm grip alone around the knee is enough to perform this stretch.**

Chapter 8:
Travel Stretches

- **Neck Rolls**
  - -The ideal position for this is seated due to the position itself isolating the neck and upper back muscles. Alternatively, you can perform this standing, but let's say you're in a moving vehicle, your safety is more important, your space is limited, and balance may be required. First, sit in a chair that has back support and position yourself in an upright posture. Next, same as the ankle circles, pretend you are trying to draw a circle in front of you with your chin. Perform slowly.
  - -Major muscles stretched: Trapezius, SCM (sternocleidomastoids), Levator Scapulae, and Cervical Erector Spinae Muscle Groups

- **Tips:** Express caution when performing this stretch. It will be very easy to make yourself disoriented and dizzy if attempting to perform this stretch quickly. You may close your eyes in an attempt to prevent this from happening.

Chapter 8:
Travel Stretches

- **Shoulder Rolls**
  - The ideal position for this is to be seated. Alternatively, you can perform it standing, but let's say you're in a moving vehicle, your safety is more important, your space is limited, and balance may be required. First, sit in a chair that has a back to it and position yourself in an upright posture. Next, as with the ankle circles and neck rolls, pretend that you are trying to draw a circle with the sides of your shoulders. Once completed, perform on the other shoulder.
  - Major Muscles stretched: Trapezius, Levator Scapulae, Rhomboids, Pectoralis Minor, and Serratus Anterior Superior.

- Tips: Make sure to keep your neck and head in an upright position when performing this stretch. This stretch be performed on both sides at the same time or individually and in a clockwise or counterclockwise fashion.

Chapter 9: Stretch Smart - Tips From A Chiropractor

Now that we identified which stretches work best for you, let's go deeper into how to prevent these problems the best we can.

Posture will always be a topic in the chiropractic space. It is one of the most significant health contributors that many people don't focus on. Practicing good posture can help prevent body strains, enhance your breathing, and improve your body's biomechanics. There are also numerous tools at your disposal that can be used independently or in conjunction with any of the stretches in this guide.

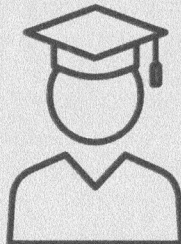

Chapter 9: Stretch Smart - Tips From A Chiropractor

- Posture Hacks:
  - Plumb Line
    - This is the ideal posture where all of the anatomical landmarks of the body are in line with each other. In other words, imagine there is a vertical line (a plumb line) going from the top of your head all the way down into your heels. These landmarks include the top of the ears, ends of the shoulders, sides of the hips, sides of the knees, and ankles.
  - Standing
    - Your standing posture should be tall, eyes looking straight, shoulders back, and feet about shoulder-width apart. If you are slouching or leaning forward, then proper posture isn't being achieved.
  - Sitting
    - Finding a seat with good back support while keeping your head looking straight and feet flat on the floor will always help in maintaining good posture. Slouching forward or leaning forward to avoid using back support is not practicing proper posture.

Chapter 9: Stretch Smart - Tips From A Chiropractor

- Desk Work
  - The same principles of sitting are applied here as well. More importantly, the top line of the computer screen that you work on should be adjusted to your eye level, adding lumbar support to your chair, and taking regular breaks every 30 minutes when possible to stand up, walk around, or stretch.
- Sleeping
  - The only two ways I have ever recommended to my patients to sleep are either on their side or on their back. If <u>sleeping on your side</u>, place a pillow in between your legs (knees and lower legs) to keep the spine in alignment, remove unwanted tension in the pelvis, and to decrease movement throughout the night. If <u>sleeping on your back</u>, put a pillow under your lower legs (under the calf muscles) to keep the spine in alignment, remove pressure on the lower back, and to decrease movement throughout the night. The one position I always advise steering clear of is sleeping on your stomach. This position compromises the spine, places unnecessary rotation in the spine, and stresses your lower back curvature.

Chapter 9: Stretch Smart - Tips From A Chiropractor

- Lifting
  - The spine is incredibly resilient to different pressures and is able to perform multiple movements at a whim. In general, lifting anything at all requires the involvement of the spine to perform an action. Unfortunately, in my practice, I see many of my patients pick up objects from the ground incorrectly. By this incorrect way, there is no utilization of the lower extremities (legs) and dependence on the lower back alone. The correct way to lift something off of the ground is as follows:
  -Stand in front of the object, looking at the object with little neck flexion, bending the knees while keeping the spine straight to engage the object, feet flat on the ground, grabbing the object with both hands and arms, placing the object close to your body and using the strength of your legs to lift to the object up.

Chapter 9: Stretch Smart - Tips From A Chiropractor

- Recommended tools for stretching and daily pain relief:
  - Foam Roller
    - It is a cylindrical tool used for self-myofasical release. Myofascia is the connective tissue between muscle layers and other soft tissues. Think of it like glue!
    - It is effective for releasing muscle knots, improving blood flow in the tissue you're rolling it on, and recovery in post-workout routines. Imagine it's like a form of self-massage.
  - Safety Tips: Foam Rollers are meant to go over broad, muscles and skin. Avoid rolling over certain areas with little soft tissue such as the knee joint and sides of the hip joint. Just like the stretches listed in previous chapters, do slow controlled movements and breathe. Avoid using the Foam Roller over open wounds, open fractures, areas of skin irritation or conditions, and areas affected by underlying diseases.
  - Bonus Tip: You can use this alongside the stretches you perform. For example, in the figure four stretch, you can first perform the stretch itself then use the foam roller right after, and vice versa.

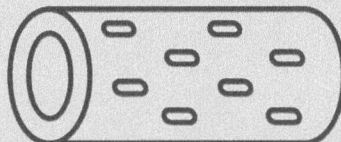

Chapter 9: Stretch Smart - Tips From A Chiropractor

- Lacrosse Ball
  - It is a firm rubber ball that is, as the name says, used for the sport of Lacrosse.
  - Surprisingly, it doubles a great tool for working on muscle knots and trigger points. It would be best to use it against a wall or the floor. Remember that these irritations develop over time. Using the lacrosse ball over those irritations to obtain relief will take time.
- Safety Tip: These spots are hyper-irritable meaning the pain can be intense when certain pressure is applied. Start by using pressure with your index and middle finger to gauge how much pressure can be tolerated. You can then graduate to using the lacrosse ball. Avoid using the Lacrosse Ball over open wounds, open fractures, areas of skin irritation or conditions, and areas that are compromised due to any underlying diseases.
- Bonus Tip: You can use this alongside the stretches you perform. For example, in the crossed-legged side bend, you can use the lacrosse ball after to release the muscle knots and trigger points that are still present.

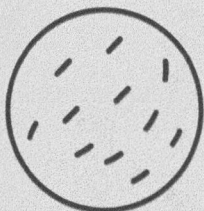

Chapter 9: Stretch Smart - Tips From A Chiropractor

○ Dry/Moist Hot Packs and Ice Packs
  ▪ Hot and Ice packs come in many different forms. The traditional heating pads you find in stores are of the dry type. Moist Hot packs usually have a foam layer or a way to retain water to provide heat and moisture to the body at the same time. Ice packs usually come in one form, they are flat and are a bit heavy because of fluid being retained inside.
  ▪ Dry/Moist Hot Packs are great for acute, subacute, and chronic conditions. This includes prolonged muscle soreness (after injury or days after an intense workout), chronic muscle pain, chronic muscle tightness, and chronic muscle stiffness. Ice packs are best for new acute injuries and inflammation (initial 24-72 hours). This includes immediate post-workout soreness, injury after a fall, and any immediate physical traumas to the body.
  ▪ My typical recommendation that I give in practice is to perform these self-therapies for 15-20 minutes as many times as possible a day.

Chapter 9: Stretch Smart - Tips From A Chiropractor

- ○ Safety Tip: Wrap a towel around any of the packs as a safety barrier between you and the pack. Intense temperatures may cause hypersensitivity or burns. Avoid using the Dry/Moist Hot Packs over open wounds, open fractures, areas of skin irritation or conditions, and areas that are compromised due to any underlying diseases.
- ○ Bonus Tip: Use any of the types of packs before bed to get a better night's sleep.

Chapter 9: Stretch Smart - Tips From A Chiropractor

- TENS/EMS unit
  - Transcutaneous Electrical Nerve Stimulation (TENS) and Electrical Muscle Stimulation (EMS) devices have been around for several decades now. The former is used for pain relief and the latter is used to stimulate and strengthen muscles.
  - These units are good for short-term pain relief in the muscles and joints and to strengthen muscles that need to be re-educated after an injury or episodes of weakness.
  - It is best used for post-workout routines, chronic pain, long days of physical work, and even before stretching tight muscles.

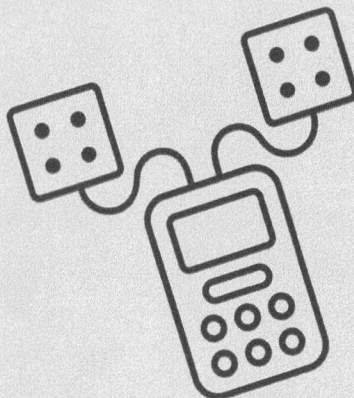

Chapter 9: Stretch Smart - Tips From A Chiropractor

- Safety Tip: Every TENS/EMS unit has different modes and intensities that range from relaxing to more stimulating. As a general rule of thumb, start with the most relaxing mode possible and start with minimal intensity until you are ready to tolerate stronger levels. Perform this self-therapy at most for 15-20 minutes, 1-3 times a day. Due to continuous or pulsed muscle contraction, it is almost like replicating a workout, so be advised you may be sore after prolonged use. Avoid using the TENS/EMS unit over open wounds, open fractures, areas of skin irritation or conditions, and areas that are compromised due to any underlying diseases.
- Bonus Tip: You can use the Dry/Moist Hot Pack or Ice Pack over the pads of the TENS/EMS unit to perform two simultaneous therapies for additional relief.

Chapter 9: Stretch Smart - Tips From A Chiropractor

○ Lumbosacral support belt
  - These belts can range from a single flexible band to upgraded ones that have flexible back plates and tightening straps.
  - These belts offer great support for lumbosacral pain and lumbosacral conditions. Their general purpose is to limit the range of motion to the lower back (never to fully restrict ROM).
  - Best used for chronic lumbosacral pain, performing chores around your home, and situations where you know you will be sitting/standing for more than 20 minutes continuously.

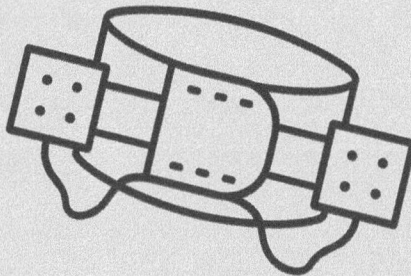

Chapter 9: Stretch Smart - Tips From A Chiropractor

○ **Safety Tip: Do not wear this belt continuously. The more you restrict your lower back from natural movement, the more dependent you'll be to wear the belt. In other words, your muscles can become weak if they're not given a break. In practice, my typical recommendation is to wear the belt if you're standing, sitting, or lifting for more than 20 minutes. The maximum amount of time I typically suggest wearing the belt would be 1 hour to 1.5 hours, taking the belt off for 15-20 minutes, performing the stretches as I listed in this guide for the lower back, and then placing the belt back on for continued relief for the rest of the day. If your belt has tightening straps, make sure to tighten them to where it feels snug and firm over the abdomen and back. If the compression is strong or if it's tight to the point where you cannot breathe, then this means that the fitting is incorrect. Please do not wear the belt to perform exercise unless the belt manufacturer specifically states this as a feature. Do not sleep with the belt on.**

Chapter 9: Stretch Smart - Tips From A Chiropractor

Avoid using the lumbosacral support belt over open wounds, fractures, areas of skin irritation or conditions, and areas that are compromised due to any underlying diseases. Do not use the belt on bare skin.

- Bonus Tip: If your Dry/Moist Hot Pack or Ice Pack is thin enough, you can attempt to place it in the back of the belt to experience the relief you need and the belt will keep the pack in place

Chapter 9: Stretch Smart - Tips From A Chiropractor

- Consistency and Tracking
  - I often find myself reminding my patients that 'Rome wasn't built in a day.' Stretching will not be an overnight fix. Instead, what it will do is lessen muscle aches, reduce stiffness, improve your posture, regulate and improve blood flow, aid in the prevention of injury, and help with physical and mental health.
  - As I mentioned at the beginning of this guide, there are 24 hours, 1440 minutes, and 86,400 seconds in a day. It will take no longer than 15 minutes to stretch your body throughout the day. You can absolutely mix and match what works best for you and skip what doesn't work for you. Doing stretches daily will always be best, but the more consistent you are with your personalized routine, the sooner your body will thank you.

Chapter 9: Stretch Smart - Tips From A Chiropractor

○ Tracking
  ▪ Calendar (Physical/Digital)
    -On your fridge or desk
    -On your smartphone
  ▪ Apps
    -Calendar app on iPhone or Android
    -Reminder app on iPhone
    -Google Calendar
    -Habitica
    -Loop Habit Tracker (Android)
    -TickTick: To-Do List
  ▪ Journal
    -Making a journal can be very beneficial. You can have a more detailed view of what stretches you performed, for how long, how many sets and reps you were able to do, and make benchmarks for the next session.

Chapter 9: Stretch Smart - Tips From A Chiropractor

o Benchmarks
   -It would be worth noting what stretches
    felt tolerable, which stretches felt challenging,
    which stretches helped your body the most,
    and setting goals.
   -Goal setting can include increasing flexibility
    of muscle, improving range of motion, and
    decreasing levels of pain.
   ▪ Short Term: 1-4 weeks
      • Examples: Stretching every day for 5
        minutes, holding a stretch for 30
        seconds, adding a piece of equipment
        (like a foam roller) into your routine, etc.
   ▪ Long Term 1-3 months
      • Being able to touch your toes, reducing
        low back tension after work, being able
        to rise out of bed with 50% or less pain,
        etc.

Chapter 9: Stretch Smart - Tips From A Chiropractor

○ Pairing with a Routine
  - If you're a multitasker, or just the type of person who likes to do two things at the same time, then let's show some scenarios where you can pair a task with stretching.
    ▪ Pair brushing your teeth with:
      • Sustained Neck Stretches (Ch.3)
      • Crossed Leg Side Bending Stretch (Ch.7)
      • Standing Sustained Quad Stretch (Ch.5)
      • Sustained calf stretch (Ch.5)
    ▪ Pair watching TV with:
      • Sustained Neck Stretches
      • Bending down to touch toes (Ch.5)
      • Child's Pose (Ch.6)
      • Piriformis Stretch (aka Figure Four Stretch, Ch.7)
    ▪ Pair with waiting on hold for a phone call
      • Child's Pose
      • Neck Rolls (Ch.8)
      • Shoulder Rolls (Ch.8)
      • Wrist ROM (Ch.4)
    ▪ Everyone has different routines so think of what you do regularly and how you can incorporate stretches into it.

Chapter 9: Stretch Smart - Tips From A Chiropractor

- ○ Celebration and Reflection
  - ▪ You've hit an important milestone for your health. You worked towards decreasing pain in your body while also improving your posture, flexibility, and mobility! Remember, this is all a slow build towards something greater for your future.
  - ▪ Recognize that the information you absorbed while reading this pocket guide matters to improving your overall wellbeing. Some questions you should be asking yourself:

    -How do I feel different in my body?

    -Did stretching get easier over time?

    -Has my pain or stiffness decreased?

    -Was I consistent and how can I continue to be consistent?

    -What was easy? What was hard?

    -What are my next goals I want to achieve?

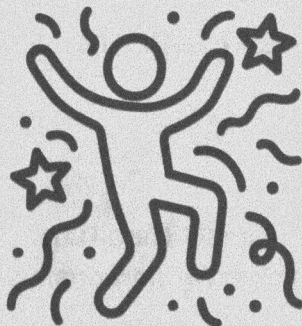

Chapter 9: Stretch Smart - Tips From A Chiropractor

- Treat yourself to something for your accomplishments. This can be anything at all! Such as getting a new piece of equipment, verbal praise for yourself ("I stretched at least three times this week!"), having a favorite snack, dedicating extra time to your favorite hobby or share your progress with a family member/friend.
- Affirmations
  -Create a personalized affirmation for yourself that centers around who you are, what goals you're achieving and envisioning your future.
- Here is a template that you can use each month for reflection.
  -My favorite stretch:
  -Most noticeable improvement:
  -One thing I'm proud of:
  -New goal for next month:

See Page 97 for a full stretch tracker for personal use

Chapter 10: A Close and Disclaimer (Fun!)

Thank you first and foremost for taking your time to explore my guide and making a huge investment to your body's health. Whether you are just starting your wellness journey or you're already deep into it, just remember that you are a powerful human being that can tackle emotional, physical and mental hardships head on. Stretching is a key motivating factor to help you along the way. Maintaining consistency, patience and discipline are the biggest tools in your toolbox. Always listen to your body and your body will respond accordingly. As my mentor once said to me and applies to all aspects of life is that "sameness will kill you".

Chapter 10: A Close and Disclaimer (Fun!)

Remember: Stretching is not a quick fix. It is all about progress. Celebrate every small win you have and reflect on how far you've come. If you ever feel like you're falling behind or off track, just realize it isn't the end. You are always able to begin again. The purpose of this guide is to give you a foundation you can use anytime, anywhere.

Stay strong, stay mobile, and keep stretching towards your best self.

Yours in Health,
Dr. Michael A. Martinez

Chapter 10: A Close and Disclaimer (Fun!)

Disclaimer:

This stretch guide is intended for general educational and informational purposes only. It is not a substitute for professional medical advice, diagnosis, or treatment. Always consult with your physician, chiropractor, physical therapist, or other qualified healthcare provider before beginning any new stretching or exercise program — especially if you have existing injuries, health conditions, or concerns.

The author and publisher disclaim any liability for injury or loss sustained directly or indirectly from the use of this guide. Perform all stretches safely and within your comfort level. If you experience pain, dizziness, or shortness of breath while stretching, stop immediately and seek medical advice.

Your health is your responsibility. This guide is here to support you — not replace personalized care.

Anatomy of a Stretcher

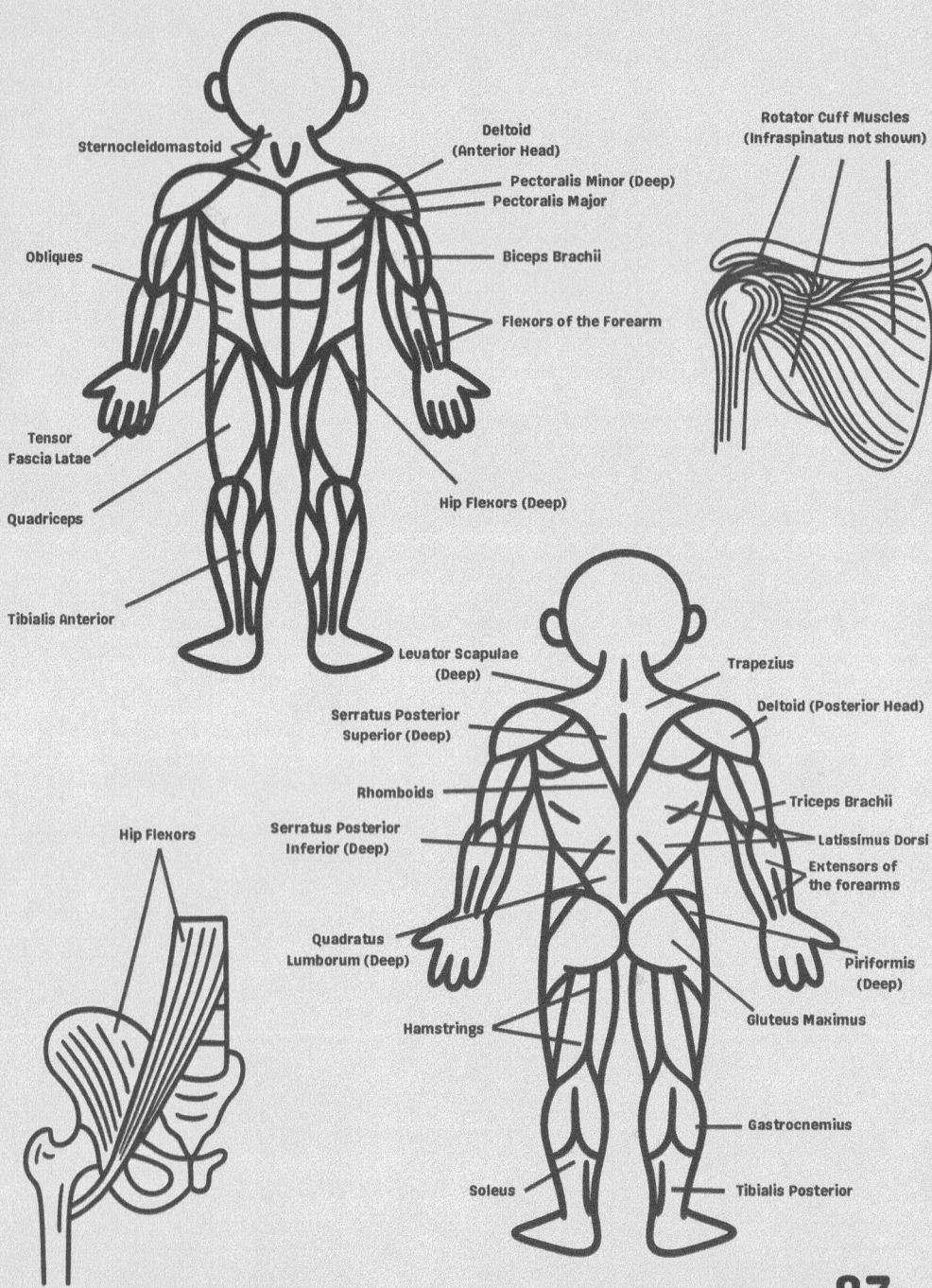

Sternocleidomastoid

Deltoid
(Anterior Head)

Pectoralis Minor (Deep)
Pectoralis Major

Biceps Brachii

Flexors of the Forearm

Obliques

Tensor
Fascia Latae

Quadriceps

Tibialis Anterior

Hip Flexors (Deep)

Rotator Cuff Muscles
(Infraspinatus not shown)

Levator Scapulae
(Deep)

Serratus Posterior
Superior (Deep)

Rhomboids

Serratus Posterior
Inferior (Deep)

Hip Flexors

Quadratus
Lumborum (Deep)

Hamstrings

Trapezius

Deltoid (Posterior Head)

Triceps Brachii

Latissimus Dorsi

Extensors of
the forearms

Piriformis
(Deep)

Gluteus Maximus

Gastrocnemius

Soleus

Tibialis Posterior

87

Glossary

- **Abduction:** Movement away from the midline of your body
- **Abrasions:** Superficial skin scrapes
- **Acute:** Sudden and short-term
- **Adduction:** Movement toward midline
- **Affirmation:** Positive self-statement
- **Anatomical Landmarks:** Body reference points
- **Biomechanics:** Movement mechanics of body
- **Benchmark:** Standard for comparison
- **Bone Spurs:** Bony growths at joints
- **Cervical Spine:** Neck portion of spine
- **Celebration:** Marking a success or goal
- **Chronic:** Long-term or recurring
- **Combined:** Two or more together
- **Compression:** Pressing or squeezing force
- **Conditions:** Health or functional states
- **Consistency:** Repeating behavior regularly
- **Contraindications:** Reasons to avoid treatment
- **Controlled:** Managed or deliberate
- **Controlled Articular Rotation:** Active joint movement drill
- **Decompress:** Reduce pressure or tension
- **Disoriented:** Confused or not alert
- **Dorsiflexion:** Toes move toward shin
- **Dynamic stretching:** Controlled movements that stretch muscles

Glossary

- **Ecchymosis:** Bruising under theskin
- **Eversion:** Sole turns outward
- **Extension:** Straightening a joint
- **Extremities:** Arms and legs
- **External Rotation:** Rotating away from center
- **Fatigue:** Tiredness or reduced performance
- **Fascia:** Connective tissue wrapping muscles
- **Flexibility:** Ability to lengthen muscles
- **Flexion:** Bending a joint
- **Force:** Strength or energy exerted
- **Forefoot:** Front part of the foot
- **Fractures:** Broken bones
- **Goals:** Desired outcomes
- **Hematomas:** Swollen blood collection
- **Hormone:** Chemical body messenger
- **Hyper Irritable:** Extremely sensitive/tender
- **Hyper-mobilizes:** Excessive joint movement
- **Ideal:** Best or optimal
- **Immobility:** Inability to move
- **Inflammation:** Swelling and irritation
- **Instability:** Lack of control or support
- **Interlocking:** Fitting or joining together
- **Internal Rotation:** Rotating toward center
- **Inversion:** Sole turns inward
- **Joint:** Connection between bones

Glossary

- **Lacerations:** Deepskin cuts
- **Lactic Acid:** Byproduct of intense activity
- **Lateral Flexion:** Side bending motion
- **Left Lower Quadrant (LLQ):** Bottom left area from your point of view
- **Left Upper Quadrant (LUQ):** Top left area from your point of view
- **Long Term:** Extended time frame
- **Lordosis:** Excessive lower back curve
- **Lower Left Quadrant:** Left lower abdomen area
- **Lower Right Quadrant:** Right lower abdomen area
- **Lumbosacral:** Lower back and sacrum
- **Lumbar Spine:** Lower back region
- **Melatonin:** Sleep-regulating hormone
- **Micro-tears:** Tiny muscle fiber damage
- **Milestone:** Significant progress point
- **Mobilize:** Make movable
- **Mobility:** Ability to move freely
- **Moderate:** Medium intensity or degree
- **Multitasking:** Doing several things simultaneously
- **Muscle Knots:** Tight muscle fiber clusters
- **Nerve Stimulation:** Activating nerves therapeutically

Glossary

- **Obstructions:** Blocksor barriers
- **Open Wounds:** Exposed tissue injuries
- **Position:** Body's placement or stance
- **Post Workout:** After exercise session
- **Post-Activity:** Following an activity
- **Posture:** Body alignment and position
- **Power:** Strength over time
- **Pre-Activity:** Before physical effort
- **Progressively:** Gradually increasing
- **Pronation:** Palm or foot turns downward
- **Radial Deviation:** Wrist bends toward thumb
- **Range of Motion (ROM):** Joint movement capability
- **Recovery:** Returning to normal state
- **Reflection:** Thoughtful review
- **Repetitions:** Times an action is repeated
- **Right Lower Quadrant (RLQ):** Bottom right area from your point of view
- **Right Upper Quadrant (RUQ):** Top right area from your poont of view
- **Routine:** Regular practice or schedule
- **Scenario:** Specific situation or context
- **Sets:** Groupings of repetitions
- **Shallow Breathing:** Low, minimal breaths

Glossary

- **Short Term:** Brief time period
- **Soft Tissue:** Muscles, tendons, ligaments
- **Soreness:** Muscle discomfort post-use
- **Spine:** Backbone structure
- **Static stretching:** Holding a stretch without movement
- **Stiffness:** Reduced movement ease
- **Strength:** Ability to exert force
- **Subacute:** Between acute and chronic
- **Supination:** Palm or foot turns upward
- **Sustained:** Held for a duration
- **Therapy:** Treatment for recovery
- **Thoracic Spine:** Mid-back region
- **Tracking:** Monitoring progress
- **Trauma:** Injury from external force
- **Transcutaneous:** Through the skin
- **Trigger Points:** Sensitive muscle spots
- **Uncontrolled:** Lacking regulation
- **Ulnar Deviation:** Wrist bends toward pinky
- **Upper Left Quadrant:** Left upper abdomen
- **Upper Right Quadrant:** Right upper abdomen
- **Warm-Up:** Prepares body for activity
- **Yoga:** Flexibility and breathing practice

QR Codes for all stretches are found at the end of the book

Suggested Reading

This guide is informed by clinical experience and best practices in physical medicine. For further reading, consult the following publications....

Behm, David G et al. "Acute effects of muscle stretching on physical performance, range of motion, and injury incidence in healthy active individuals: a systematic review." Applied physiology, nutrition, and metabolism = Physiologie appliquee, nutrition et metabolisme vol. 41,1 (2016): 1-11. doi:10.1139/apnm-2015-0235

Page, Phil. "Current concepts in muscle stretching for exercise and rehabilitation." International journal of sports physical therapyvol. 7,1 (2012): 109-19.

American College of Sports Medicine (ACSM). (2022). ACSM's Guidelines for Exercise Testing and Prescription (11th ed.). Wolters Kluwer.

Konrad, A., & Tilp, M. (2014). Increased Range of Motion after Static Stretching is Not Due to Changes in Muscle and Tendon Structures. Clinical Biomechanics, 29(6), 636–642. https://doi.org/10.1016/j.clinbiomech.2014.04.013

McHugh, M. P., & Cosgrave, C. H. (2010). To Stretch or Not to Stretch: The Role of Stretching in Injury Prevention and Performance. Scandinavian Journal of Medicine & Science in Sports, 20(2), 169–181. https://doi.org/10.1111/j.1600-0838.2009.01058.x

Nelson, R. T. (2006). A Comparison of the Immediate Effects of Static Stretching and Dynamic Stretching on Hip Range of Motion. Journal of Strength and Conditioning Research, 20(4), 819–823. https://doi.org/10.1519/R-18135.1

Suggested Reading

Shrier, I. (2004). Does Stretching Improve Performance? A
   Systematic and Critical Review of the Literature. Clinical Journal
   of Sport Medicine, 14(5), 267–273.
   https://doi.org/10.1097/00042752-200409000-00005

Alter, M. J. (2004). Science of Flexibility (3rd ed.). Human Kinetics.

Cervical Range of Motion

Thoracic Range of Motion

Lumbar Range of Motion

Combined Cervical ROM

Combined Thoracic ROM

Combined Lumbar ROM

Shoulders Range of Motion

Combined Shoulder ROM

Hips Range of Motion

Hips Combined ROM - Hip CARs

Ankles Range of Motion

Ankles Combined ROM

Wrists Range of Motion

Wrists Combined Range of Motion

Wall Stretch

Standing (or Side Lying) Quad Stretch

Sitting Hamstring Stretch

Calf Wall Stretch

One Legged Lunge Stretch (Sustained)

Child's Pose

Legs Up the Wall Pose

Corpse Pose

Leg Swings

Arm Circles	One Legged Lunge Stretch (Dynamic)	Lunging Hip Flexor Stretch
Piriformis Stretch aka Figure Four Stretch	Cross Legged Side Bend	Ankle Circles
Knee Hug	Shoulder Rolls	Neck Rolls

If you have any comments, questions, or difficulty
in accessing the videos, please search for the
YouTube playlist with the same name as the guide
or email me at dcmichaelmartinez@gmail.com

Stretch Tracker

Stretch Tracker: Weekly Progress Log

Day	Morning Mobilizer	Desk Relief	Post Workout	Evening Wind-Down	Travel Notes
Monday	☐	☐	☐	☐	☐
Tuesday	☐	☐	☐	☐	☐
Wednesday	☐	☐	☐	☐	☐
Thursday	☐	☐	☐	☐	☐
Friday	☐	☐	☐	☐	☐
Saturday	☐	☐	☐	☐	☐
Sunday	☐	☐	☐	☐	☐

Notes can include questions on Page 82

Special Thanks

Natalie Herman

Sarah Jacobs

Carlos & Maria Martinez

Edward Benavides

Mark Ason

Drew Knox

Andres Rodriguez

Michael Sofer

Author's Note

Stretching is one of those things we all know we should do—but it's usually the first thing to get pushed aside. I've seen it in my patients and I've felt it myself. Over the years, I realized that people aren't skipping it because they're lazy—they're skipping it because they're overwhelmed, unsure, or just don't know where to start. I created Go Stretch Yourself! to change that. This guide is meant to be simple, practical, and real. No fluff. No pressure. Just the kind of stretches I've seen help people feel looser, lighter, and more in control of how their body moves and feels. Whether you're trying to wake up without stiffness, reset after a long drive, or wind down from a stressful day, you'll find something in here that meets you where you are. You don't need to be flexible to start—you just need to start. Thanks for trusting me to be part of your routine. I hope this little book helps you move better, breathe deeper, and feel more at home in your body.

— Dr. Michael Martinez

www.ingramcontent.com/pod-product-compliance
Lightning Source LLC
Chambersburg PA
CBHW060511280326
41933CB00014B/2928